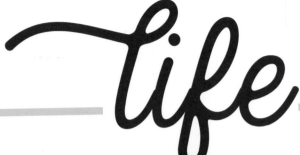

life

UNPLUGGED

RESET · RELAX · RECONNECT

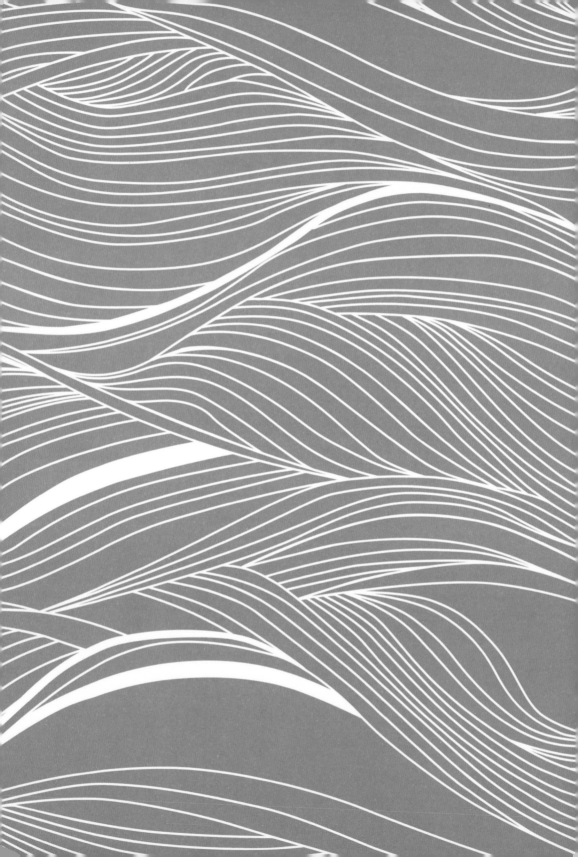

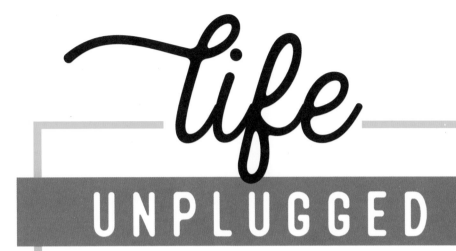

life

UNPLUGGED

RESET · RELAX · RECONNECT

A DIGITAL DETOX WORKBOOK

MELEAH BOWLES & ELISE WILLIAMS RIKARD

ROCK
POINT

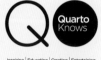

First published in 2019 by Rock Point,
an imprint of The Quarto Group
142 West 36th Street, 4th Floor
New York, NY 10018 USA
T (212) 779-4972 F (212) 779-6058
WWW.QUARTOKNOWS.COM

Rock Point titles are also available at discount for retail, wholesale, promotional, and bulk purchase. For details, contact the Special Sales Manager by email at specialsales@quarto.com or by mail at The Quarto Group, Attn: Special Sales Manager, 100 Cummings Center, Suite 265D, Beverly, MA 01915, USA.

10 9 8 7 6 5 4 3 2 1

ISBN: 978-1-63106-673-3

Publisher: Rage Kindelsperger
Managing Editor: Cara Donaldson
Editor: Keyla Pizarro-Hernández
Cover and Interior Design: Katie Cooper

Printed in China

DEDICATION

For Katie, our designer and our third set of eyes.

—Elise and Meleah

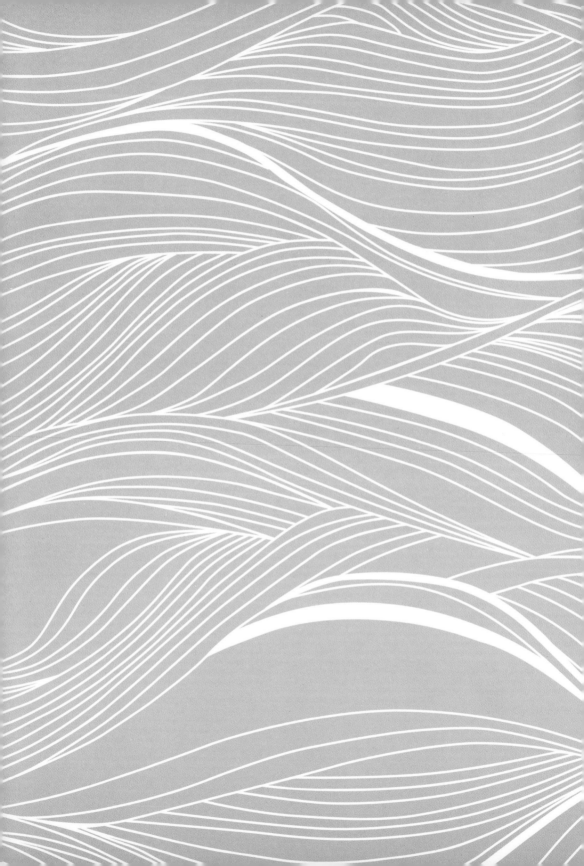

TABLE OF

contents

Introduction

Meleah and Elise here! We're best friends, writers, editors, social media addicts, and TV-bingeing junkies. You could say technology is a pretty big part of every aspect of our lives. When we first heard about digital detoxing, we were not on board. We thought, "Well, we aren't addicted to our phones, social media, or any of that, so why bother detoxing?" Our phones aren't hurting anything, right?

We like getting our Monday-night TV fix. We like playing video games. We like keeping up with the latest celebrity news online. And honestly, how on earth could we completely unplug and take a "timeout" from everything and everyone? What did people even do before phones were smart and Netflix was a standard way to spend a Friday night?

But then we realized that's exactly the point—and maybe technology is harming us after all. The constant connection is literally messing with our brains. Being connected 24/7 honestly sounds like a good thing. You can answer every email the moment it hits your inbox. You can always check in on a friend and have a virtual chat. You can always keep up with the latest news, getting real-time updates on every single crisis.

The bad news is, staying tethered to your electronics means you never have time to shut down your brain. Filling every spare moment with chatter—even with friends—leaves our lives lacking silence. Witnessing everything that goes on in the world and trying to care about every single cause is honestly exhausting and emotionally draining. After all, we're only human. While it's good to care about and help others, some days all you can do is come home after work and feed yourself. And that's okay!

From a self-esteem standpoint, it stands to reason that comparing yourself to every perfect selfie, every snapshot of someone's life or lifestyle blog is just fuel for the critical voice in your head. As far as our relationships with each other go, if we're spending all of our time binge-watching, then we aren't spending time with our friends.

By this point, unlike celebrity-endorsed detox tea (we've tried them—they're not tasty and the side effects are... unpleasant), a digital detox sounds kind of nice, right? We think so, and while writing this book, we spoke to several therapists and digital detox experts who think so too. You'll get their tips and advice on breaking the digital cycle (as well as our own) and also a few challenges we put together for you along the way!

SO PUT DOWN THE PHONE,

TURN OFF THE TV, AND

pay attention.

Digtal Detox Defined

Open Facebook and someone is either getting engaged or sharing opinions no one asked for. Scroll through your Instagram feed and that one girl from high school is promoting the latest multi-level marketing product and bragging about her "hustle." Pop over to Twitter and you'll be bombarded with celebrities yelling at other celebrities for not doing (read: tweeting) enough to solve the world's problems.

It never seems to slow down or get less frustrating. (Not that it stops us from logging in, of course.) Some days, all the technology can start to feel, well, toxic. And when something is toxic, the best thing to do is take a break.

For this particular technological toxicity, we're proposing a "digital detox." Digital detox means different things to different people. For some, it means completely unplugging from everything digital—your phone, your tablet, your TV, your video games, your laptop, everything. For others? It can be taking social media out of their daily routine or simply spending less time on their phone.

Digital detoxing, the way we see it, is taking a break from your digital reality to focus more on your actual reality. As with any detox, you'll be ridding yourself of toxins—in this case, digital toxins—to become a happier, healthier person.

The hope is that once you've purged yourself of these digital toxins, you'll be able to more clearly understand the effect that technology is having on you personally, as well as get chores done that you've been neglecting, and ultimately learn to live more in the moment.

So why do you need a break in the first place? We're essentially all living in a collective Digital Danger Zone. There's research for days (as in, it would take literal days for us to list all of it here) demonstrating that too much technology time is bad for your mental health, your work, and your relationships.

One example is a study by Andrew K. Przybylski and Netta Weinstein published in 2012 that concluded that just having your phone near you can have "negative effects on closeness, connection, and conversation quality," interfering with your relationships as a whole. Think of the last time you went to grab lunch or coffee with a friend and they had their phone in their hand. Did you feel like you had their full attention? Or vice versa? Probably not—more likely, even if you weren't aware of it, you were wondering when one of your phones was going to vibrate.

While phones can help keep us connected to those we love who are far away, they're not so good for connecting with the people who are right in front of your face.

Phones also aren't good to have by your side when you're trying to focus. Think about the last time you worked on a project or had a deadline—how many times were you interrupted by your phone?

Technology in general functions as a distraction. If you're taking notes with your laptop, it's tempting to open a new tab and before you know it, you're off-task. On the other hand, if you're writing in a notebook, distractions are further away. Watching TV while working on a project can quickly turn into just...watching TV. That's great if your goal is to watch more TV, but not so great if you're trying to actually get things done.

And there's more where that came from.

The Center for Humane Technology has compiled conclusions from dozens of sources into a project titled

"Ledger of Harms." There were some common themes in all of this research. The main takeaways are that overuse of technology and over-immersion in the digital world has the potential to harm our attention span, mental health, relationships, and children among other things.

For example, they found that when a notification comes in, most people will check that notification within a few minutes. Even if they wait longer to check notifications, most people report feeling distracted and less able to get their focus back to the task at hand. This lack of attention negatively affects our work, productivity, and is a big reason why technology use can negatively affect relationships. Interpersonal relationships thrive when two people invest the time and attention to really listen to each other and understand the other's point of view.

And when we chatted with Life Coach, Vikki Yaffe, about the ways phones and technology affect our mental health, she confirmed that we weren't alone in being distracted by our phones. Yaffe says, "Even when there's no sound coming from the phone, there is the on-going possibility that there will be. The problem is not that technology exists, it's that we are using it 24/7." It's essentially turning us all, she says, into "one big stress time bomb."

In fact, our phones contribute to major anxiety by encouraging avoidance, disrupting sleep, and fostering a technology dependence.

AVOIDANCE COPING

When given the chance, people avoid discomfort and pain. It's human nature. So when we are faced with an awkward or uncomfortable situation, we may overindulge in things that will distract us: eating, shopping, and mindlessly scrolling through the web. It's a type of "avoidance coping," which is what psychologists would call a maladaptive coping skill, aka an unhealthy habit.

In the short term, distracting yourself with technology is great and seems to alleviate anxiety. However, Yaffe points out that it doesn't actually get rid of the discomfort. She says, "It actually feeds it, and it remains there, in the background, feeling more uncomfortable, spreading to other parts of your life and other situations, so before you know it you're watching Netflix to avoid feeling guilty about spending too much time on your phone." Avoidance is the brain's way of procrastinating your anxiety, and procrastination never works well.

SLEEP DISRUPTION

In a study conducted by the Centers for Disease Control and Prevention (CDC), researchers found that one in three adults don't get enough sleep. A good night's rest is crucial to your overall health and well-being, and sleep deprivation only worsens feelings of stress and anxiety. On the flip side, when you do actually get a good night's rest, you're better able to focus and are more productive; plus, you're more likely to be in an all-around better mood.

You've probably heard that you shouldn't watch TV in bed or look at any screens for at least an hour before bed. There's a reason this tip is everywhere—this advice is pretty sound. The blue light emitted from your phone delays the release of melatonin in your body, which severely messes with your sleep cycles (your REM cycle specifically). So if you find that being tired 24/7 has just become an inherent part of your personality, your phone and/or TV could be the culprit.

TECH DEPENDENCY

Technology is such a huge part of our day-to-day lives that you can forget how much you rely on your devices. Picture it: You've left your phone at home (or your phone battery dies.) Do you take this in stride, or do you worry about how you'll get ahold of your friends? Wondering what you will do when you need directions? It's the new normal, but that doesn't mean it's good for you.

Then there's the outrageous (and toxic) hustle culture. Everywhere you look, there's an article telling you what time the "most successful" people wake up in the morning (spoiler alert: it's early), or a motivational quote about how you should just "do what you love" and turn all of your hobbies into side hustles.

When you're consistently bombarded with these messages and comparing yourself to your friends' highlight reels, it can be easy to fall into the trap of setting unrealistic expectations for yourself—that you have to do more, hustle more, achieve more.

Rachel Anne Dine, LPC and owner of Humanitas Counseling and Consulting, LLC, cautions that especially for those who "may be anxious or struggling with their own insecurities, it can really tap into that and encourage a sense of fear that they're not doing enough with their life." She adds, "The comparison trap on social media is so real and so intense and can cause such negative sense of self."

As we've mentioned (but we are really trying to drive this one home), digital detoxing isn't just about taking a break from your smartphone or just logging off of your social media for a week. Even when you are not on social media, you're probably still using some form of digital technology.

Playing video games, binging Netflix, checking your email, or watching funny cat videos—can all be (and should be) included in a digital detox.

To succeed at anything, you need to find your "why." There are countless reasons for doing a digital detox. (The limit does not exist.) Whether you want to get better beauty rest, form deeper connections with your loved ones, or just want to learn how to live more in the moment, we're sure you have your reasons.

In addition, there are several benefits to digital detoxing, including but not limited to:

- Reduced stress and anxiety
- Enhanced focus and productivity
- Improved sleeping habits
- Heightened consciousness

On the following page, take a minute to jot down a few reasons you want to take a digital break. The important thing to remember is that there's no pressure; this is designed to be a place for you to journal and free-write.

WHY I SHOULD DETOX

....

....

....

....

....

....

....

....

....

....

....

....

....

I'M DETOXING BECAUSE...

Now, try to summarize your "why"s. These are going to be your touchstones throughout the detox.

1. ....
....
....

2. ....
....
....

3. ....
....
....

So we've covered why you need to do a digital detox, but how can it actually help you?

According to Laura Rhodes-Levin, a Licensed Marriage and Family Therapist (LMFT) who specializes in the evaluation and treatment of anxiety, depression, and trauma, a little digital detoxing can go a long way to help our minds get back to their natural state of being. She says, "The digital world has demanded the brain's attention in a way that it has never known before and is not conditioned to support." In other words, our brains need a break every now and then.

A good old-fashioned digital detox will help you to clear the brain fog and focus on creating the life you want for yourself—and unlike your favorite blogger's carefully curated Instagram aesthetic, yours is real.

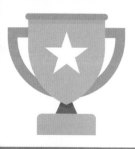

CHALLENGE

 ## STAMP SOME SNAIL MAIL

When was the last time you sent someone a card in the mail? What about a letter? It's probably been a while, and there's no time like the present. Silence your phone, turn off your TV, and grab a greeting card. If you don't have stationery on hand, you can use some printer paper or whatever you have lying around to make one. (Bonus points if you do this—it's also arts and crafts.)

Next, pick a friend or relative (or a pen pal, dealer's choice!) and just start writing. Tell them a funny story, remind them of a fun time you shared, anything. Stuff it in an envelope, scribble down their address, slap a stamp on and you're ready to go. (If you don't have their address, you can text them for it if it's one of your friends, or call your mom if it's a relative. Moms have all of the addresses.)

Tried it out? Tell us about it.

Slow & Steady

We don't believe in doing too many things at once or, in this case, giving things up cold turkey. Slow and steady always wins the race, you know.

Instead, we want to empower you to decide what you want to give up and for how long, especially for this first go-around. If you just want to give up social media for a week, do it. If you'd like to give up TV or streaming services for a month, go for it.

If you want to give up all of the above at once... well, more power to you!

Not all screen time is bad—you know what they say, everything in moderation. The moderation approach is backed up by research from The Center of Humane Technology (we mentioned them earlier) in partnership with Moment, a phone app designed to help people track their screen time.

They asked two hundred thousand iPhone users to rate how they felt after using specific apps. The findings were interesting—productivity apps and other apps that were primarily functional applications had no negative impact on mood, while social apps typically had a negative effect on mood.

Taking that a step further, the research showed that the amount of time spent on social media was a huge factor in the user-reported happiness afterwards; after about twenty minutes on Facebook, people were happier than when they spent closer to an hour online. So essentially, the less time spent on social media the happier you'll be.

But according to a 2018 report from research firm eMarketer, most people aren't just checking their notifications and then logging off. Adults (in the U.S.) spend an average of 3 hours and 35 minutes per day on mobile devices. Where do you fall? Above average, below average, or maybe somewhere in the middle? (Give it your best guess. Or use a screen-time monitoring app if you want to be sure.)

Now we'll gather some baseline data. Don't worry, this is a judgment-free zone. By documenting what your current digital habits look like, you'll be able to measure progress as you work to figure out a healthier balance. To keep things simple, when you calculate the time you spend, think about it in terms of how you spend your free time.

I USE MY...

📱 Cell Phone	....	hours/day
↖ Computer	....	hours/day
🎮 Game Console	....	hours/day
▭ Tablet	....	hours/day
🖥 TV	....	hours/day
Other	....	hours/day

Now consider how many apps you use on your phone (and/or tablet) throughout the day, and how often you're using them. Between scrolling through Facebook, trolling celebrities on Twitter, sending your BFFs memes on Instagram, texting people back, checking your personal AND work emails, planning your wedding on Pinterest, and reading fan theories about your favorite TV show, your screen time can add up pretty quickly.

Be honest with yourself—how do you feel about your relationship with technology right now? Are you able to answer a few emails and then step away from the keyboard (or put down the phone or tablet) without letting your other notifications distract you?

Or do you find yourself becoming a permanent couch cushion, with the only exercise you get from clicking "add to cart" or changing channels?

Maybe you're somewhere between those two extremes. Turn the page for a quick quiz to help you evaluate your tech use, and how it fits (or doesn't fit) into your life.

"THE FIRST STEP IS FINDING AN HOUR EACH DAY WHERE YOU FORCE YOURSELF TO GIVE UP THE SCREEN. START TEACHING YOURSELF TO IGNORE IT WHEN IT BEEPS, BUZZES OR VIBRATES. THIS IS YOUR TIME, NOT YOUR DEVICES'."

—Dr. Christopher Smithmyer, LLM

HOW BADLY DO I NEED TO DETOX?

HOW MUCH TIME DO YOU SPEND ON YOUR PHONE A DAY?

☐ Less than an hour (+1)

☐ 1-3 hours (+2)

☐ 3+ hours (+3)

HOW MUCH TIME DO YOU SPEND WATCHING TV AND MOVIES A DAY?

☐ Less than an hour (+1)

☐ 1-3 hours (+2)

☐ 3+ hours (+3)

HOW OFTEN DO PEOPLE MAKE COMMENTS ABOUT HOW MUCH TIME YOU SPEND ON YOUR PHONE?

☐ Never (+1)

☐ Sometimes (+2)

☐ Pretty often (+3)

HOW OFTEN DO YOU FIND YOURSELF ENVYING YOUR FRIENDS AND FOLLOWERS?

☐ Never (liar!) (+1)

☐ Sometimes (+2)

☐ Only when someone posts pics of their vacation...or their engagement ring...or their cute dogs... (+3)

HOW OFTEN DO YOU FIND YOURSELF WISHING THERE WERE MORE HOURS IN THE DAY?

☐ Never (liar x2!) (+1)

☐ Sometimes (+2)

☐ Only when I catch myself mindlessly scrolling through social media for hours on end or telling Netflix that yes, in fact, I do want to continue watching... (+3)

Results

(5–7 POINTS) YOU SHOULD PROBABLY DETOX

Your relationship with social media is pretty healthy! Good for you, Glen Coco. You could still benefit from a digital detox, but the good news is it'll probably be a breeze for you.

(8–10 POINTS) YOU SHOULD DEFINITELY DETOX

You could definitely benefit from doing a digital detox. Just think of how many more books you could read in the amount of time you spend scrolling through your feed!

(11–15 POINTS) START DETOXING ASAP

Simply put, digital detoxing was created with you in mind. Yes, you. You need to start your detox, like, yesterday. Your loved ones will thank us later.

If we were male CEOs who liked sports, this is where we would give a pep talk in the form of ambiguous sports metaphors. But we are not CEOs of a company, nor are we male, and we're definitely not into sports. (How do you think we got addicted to our phones in the first place?) So instead of a pep talk, we're going to get really real with you: We love our TV and we like our celebrity stalking, so a realistic game plan needs to be in place before we do anything drastic.

What are you going to do with those three-and-a-half hours a day? The time you usually spend looking at what your friends are eating could now be spent doing literally anything—reading, taking a yoga class, or even cooking your own dinner. (Unheard of, right?)

Once you take a break from what everyone else is doing with their lives, you'll be able to actually focus on your own. Check in with yourself. How do you want to spend your time? Do you actually want to jet off somewhere new every other month like your favorite Instagram hate-follow or do you want time to curl up with a good book once a week instead?

Really, we're taking this back to you finding your "why." In the last chapter, your "why" was focused on how you want to feel. Now, build on that and discover what you want to do. To put it another way, in Marie Kondo-fashion, what would spark joy in your life?

Remember earlier when we said there was going to be more journaling ahead? Grab that pencil, and get ready to journal. But don't take yourself too seriously because...

JOURNALING IS NOT A LEGALLY BINDING contract.

Journal about how you might like to spend your time. Take this space to work out your thoughts.

....

....

....

....

....

....

....

....

....

....

....

....

Now let's build on that last journaling exercise. What activities did you write about the most? Did a common theme emerge?

On the following page, turn those thoughts into action and choose three activties to focus on. They will be the cornerstone of your digital detox! By planning ahead and being deliberate about how you will use your time, you will avoid accidentally slipping into your old habits.

Whatever you decide, trust us, all those political memes and gender-reveal videos will still be there waiting for you when you get back.

I WILL SPEND MORE TIME...

1. ....
   ....
   ....

2. ....
   ....
   ....

3. ....
   ....
   ....

12 Tips for Breaking

1. TELL EVERYONE YOU KNOW SO THEY CAN HOLD YOU ACCOUNTABLE

2. TURN OFF EVERY PUSH NOTIFICATION ON YOUR PHONE AND TABLET

3. TURN OFF UNREAD FLAGS ON EMAIL.

4. TURN YOUR PHONE TO GRAYSCALE.

5. USE A SMART WATCH SO YOU ONLY READ TEXT MESSAGES, BUT DON'T SCROLL SOCIAL MEDIA.

6. CREATE A "ME" SPACE (FREE OF YOUR ELECTRONICS!)

Your Digital Habits

7. BUY AN ALARM CLOCK AND KEEP YOUR PHONE AWAY FROM YOUR BED—AND YOUR BEDROOM.

8. CREATE FAMILY/FRIEND SPACE FOR BONDING TIME.

9. CANCEL YOUR STREAMING SERVICE SUBSCRIPTIONS.

10. SWAP IN YOUR SMARTPHONE FOR AN OLD-SCHOOL FLIP PHONE.

11. LET A FRIEND BORROW YOUR GAMING CONSOLE WHILE YOU DETOX.

12. DON'T BE HARD ON YOURSELF IF YOU MESS UP. THE IMPORTANT THING IS THAT YOU'RE TRYING.

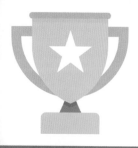

CHALLENGE

SPARK JOY FOR AN HOUR A DAY

Write down a list of 5-7 analog (that means offline) activities that make you happy—whether it's a solo activity, like reading a good book, or something more social, like wine night with your girls or taking a cooking class with your partner—and swap out an hour of phone or Netflix time each day to do something on the list. (If this doesn't turn out to be doable during the week, try changing things up and increasing the amount of time for this challenge on the weekends.)

Take it one step further and write each activity on a little scrap of paper, crumple them all up, put them in a jar, and randomly choose one each day for a week, or drop them back in the jar when you're done and keep it going longer.

Tried it out? Tell us about it.

Minimalism & Mindfulness

Minimalism and mindfulness—while they do make for a great alliteration, they're more than that. (They're also more than just trendy buzzwords.) They're the keys to a successful digital detox, and they go hand-in-hand.

There are tons of documentaries and books about minimalism, but minimalism, simply put, is about living with less. This traditionally means having less in your home; less clothing, less clutter, which means less to worry about, which leads to less stress and anxiety. The theory is that by having less stuff around to distract you, you will become more mindful—which sounds pretentious, but really just means getting in touch with your thoughts and emotions. When you master mindfulness, you'll make better decisions and spend your time in more healthy ways.

It's easy to focus on big life events, like birthdays, weddings, and graduations, because they are exciting. But life is really made up of a billion little moments between the milestones. According to Laura Rhodes-Levin, LMFT, "It is virtually impossible, pun intended, to experience and enjoy all that the world has to offer when your face is buried in your phone or a computer screen." Mindfulness connects us to the present moment.

DECLUTTERING DIGITALLY

These same concepts can be applied digitally. Think about your social media accounts—do they make you happy? Do you find yourself getting annoyed when you see a joke fifteen different times in your newsfeed?

Look at who you're including in your online life—are there ways you could curate that to make your time online less stressful? If there's a certain page or account you consistently find messes with your mood, unfollow them. If there's someone who's driving you up a wall with their random posts, consider muting them for a month or even unfollowing or unfriending them.

Now think about your email. Unless you're an inbox-zero devotee, your email could benefit from a clean out. Start by archiving anything older than ninety days. If it has been fine without your attention for three months, it doesn't need to continue to take up space in your inbox. Then use folders to group your emails, and move whatever you can there. You can also take it one step further and set up rules for your emails to automatically be sorted into the various folders you created.

For the next phase, we recommend taking action and decluttering by deleting your social media apps and/or canceling your streaming services. Without your Netflix queue calling your name and apps tethering you to your phone, you'll be less distracted by all of the notifications, messages, and memes, and be able to focus on what's actually happening around you—whether that's a cute stranger checking you out, your kid's t-ball game, your professor discussing an upcoming deadline, or just snuggle time with your pet. And without all those digital distractions, you'll be able to become more mindful with how you choose to spend your time.

TIPS FOR MAINTAINING A MINDFUL AND MINIMAL RELATIONSHIP WITH TECHNOLOGY:

 Journal, journal, journal.

Journaling can mean a dozen different things—from art journaling, to diary-style journaling, to bullet journaling. According to research on the physical act of handwriting by Anne Mangen and Jean-Luc Velay, titled "Digitizing Literacy: Reflections on the Haptics of Writing," writing by hand activates a few different processes in your brain: visual, motor, and cognitive. Keeping your brain busy reduces the temptation to attempt to multitask, and encourages you to focus on your current activity. Journaling also improves memory, increases emotional intelligence, and reduces negative feelings.

 ### Create a tech-free space.

Take it a step further and remove technology from an entire room of your home. No TV, no chargers, no gaming consoles—you get the point. Use this room as your digital-free retreat; cuddle your furbaby, turn a window into a reading nook, write in a journal, take up a new hobby like knitting, or turn the space into your own personal gym!

 ### Practice meditation.

Meditation is a great way to build your mindfulness muscles—when you learn how to clear out the daily stresses and negative thoughts from your mind, you train your brain to let that ish go.

"THE BEST PLACE TO DETOX IS YOUR OWN PERSONAL LIBRARY. IT FORCES YOU TO USE YOUR IMAGINATION AND NOT RELY ON THE VISUALIZATIONS OF OTHERS."

–Dr. Christopher Smithmyer, LLM

If you've never meditated before, you might try a meditation book, app, or a YouTube video to teach you the basics. If you already know what you're doing, set a timer each day and let your daily stresses melt away. Even if you only have ten minutes, a little meditation can go a long way.

Meditation is also a good practice for whenever you feel the urge to "plug in" because it helps refocus your energy on you, not your tech.

 Declutter your physical life.

Once you've decluttered your digital life (make sure to delete your social apps and clean up your DVR), declutter in real life as well. Donate old clothes, open that last lone box since that's been sitting there since you moved, clear off your desk space, throw away dried-up pens (I know they're your favorite, sorry!), just get rid of STUFF. It's almost as distracting as your phone!

A cluttered physical space can also keep you from enjoying and relaxing in your home. If you don't love your home base space, you're more likely to be tempted to distract yourself with technology.

 Make waking up and falling asleep a digital-free zone.

Resist the urge to grab your phone when you first wake up. Lie there for a few minutes, stretch, meditate, journal, or write down your dreams. At night, practice gratitude and write down one good thing that happened that day. Really use your time in bed (both morning and night) to check in with yourself.

Ideally, your phone won't even be stored in your bedroom at night. Revolutionary, we know.

 Get your loved ones on board.

Instead of snapping selfies with your mimosas at brunch, have all of your friends put their phones in their purses. Make the dinner table a phone-free zone by having everyone leave their phones in a different room. (Or be a *cool mom* and get a bucket just for the occasion.) If your crew won't get on board the detox train themselves, ask them to hold you accountable and help you stay offline.

 Write letters.

Letter writing is similar to journaling because, like we've covered above, the physical act of writing tricks the brain into feeling calmer and more focused. That said, letter writing gets a section all on its own because this tip is especially helpful for those who use social media specifically to stay connected with friends and family who are far away.

Instead of sharing the dirty details of your life with your five hundred followers you don't really even care about, write them down just for the people you love. (You'll need stamps, though...just in case you've never done this before!) Not only will it make you feel better, it will make them feel special to recieve a hand-written letter. It's the thought that counts.

 ### Connect for real.

Scrolling through your phone is a habit (a bad one at that), so when you find yourself reaching for your phone, send a quick text to someone to tell them you love them. (Bonus points for calling someone!) Or just put your phone somewhere out of sight so you can't easily reach for it when you feel the urge.

 ### Do things that make you forget about your phone.

Try out gardening, take a cooking class, start crocheting, or take up yoga. Grab drinks with friends. Take a cooking class. Read a really good book. Host a book club! And believe it or not, it *is* possible to have fun at a concert without recording the whole thing. (Plus, no one thinks it's as cool as you do, we promise.)

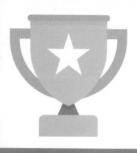

CHALLENGE

 WINE AND DINE YOURSELF

When you beat your friends to a restaurant, you probably grab a table and immediately turn to your phone while you wait. Same. We all focus on our tech to avoid downtime, boredom, and awkward social interactions, but it turns out we're using our cell phones to shield ourselves from the discomfort of being on our own.

Step outside of your comfort zone and plan a date with yourself one night. Think you can't spend thirty minutes without a distraction from your own company? Start small and try to be open to new conversations—maybe with your server, maybe with someone at the table next to you, or someone admiring the same art at a museum as you—and get to know someone you should stay on good terms with: yourself. Plus, don't underestimate the people-watching potential.

Tried it out? Tell us about it.

....

....

....

....

....

....

....

....

....

....

....

....

....

Optimizing Your Offline Options

Just like any habit or addiction you try to break or change, quitting cold turkey isn't a great gameplan. Instead, to really set yourself up for success, strive to form a new, better habit to replace the old one.

When are you the most plugged in? Could you just unplug? For example, let's say your after-work routine looks something like this: walk in your door after work, change into comfier clothes, click on the TV, pat your pet on the head, pop dinner in the microwave, and then scroll through social media for "just a minute" (aka: for at least the next hour). What does that routine look like if you just cut out the TV in the background, or set your phone down?

You could try replacing TV with your favorite playlist or podcast for an hour while you take the time to cook dinner. Or remove technology from the situation altogether and cook with your partner or invite a friend over to help you. When you make these changes with intention, you're cultivating your relationship with yourself, strengthening your relationship to your body, and just all-around probably going to feel better about yourself.

There are most likely a million things on your to-do list that get neglected because you just "don't have the time." Or maybe your reading list keeps piling up. Or maybe you just wish you had time to call your loved ones more often.

I AM HAPPY WHEN...

In the provided space below, jot down several things that make you happy.

1. ....
....

2. ....
....

3. ....
....

If you're drawing a blank, don't worry; you know we have a few examples for you! Here are a few productive ways to spend your newfound, digital-free, free time.

GO OUTSIDE

It's the refrain of parents and grandparents everywhere: kids just don't spend time outside making mud pies and playing with sticks like they used to because everyone— kids included—are glued to screens 24/7. But honestly, whatever kids these days are or aren't doing outside, most adults don't get enough vitamin D either.

According to the Environmental Protection Agency, the average American spends 87% of their life indoors (An additional 6% of time is spent in automobiles BTW, which does not count as being "outdoors"). That leaves a whopping 7% of time spent outside. And according to studies conducted by the Journal of Environmental Science and Technology, getting outside for as little as five minutes at a time improves mood and self-esteem.

So what are we DOING? There's a whole world out there! There are beaches to drink margs on, birds to hear chirping, butterflies to chase, trails to hike, pool parties to be had.

Try Out Forest Bathing

What is "forest bathing"? (Disclaimer: You do not need a bathing suit or a towel to go forest bathing. In this case, "bathing" is used to mean letting yourself be immersed in nature.)

Amos Clifford, founder of the Association of Nature and Forest Therapy Guides and Programs and author of *Your Guide to Forest Bathing: Experience the Healing Power of Nature*, calls forest bathing "a practice of connecting to nature through our senses."

Basically, take a walk in nature somewhere. It sounds simple (and it is!), but there are real health benefits. The origin of the practice has been traced back to a Japanese technique called Shinrin-yoku, which was developed in the 1980s as a response to an overworked community. Multiple studies since then have shown that practicing forest therapy results in lower blood pressure, a healthier heart rate, reduced stress, and possibly even a boosted immune system.

In her book, *The Joy of Forest Bathing: Reconnect With Wild Places & Rejuvenate Your Life*, author and certified forest guide Melanie Choukas-Bradley recommends choosing a space close to your home, adopting it as your "wild home," and visiting this place regularly for your forest bathing sessions.

When choosing your "wild home," a forest, obviously, is one option, but despite the name, you don't have to be in an actual forest to practice forest bathing. You can quite literally stop and smell the roses anywhere—while walking in your own neighborhood, visiting a city park, or planting your own garden. As long as your surroundings have a diverse environment that engages all of your senses with the color of the flora, sounds of wildlife, and smells of nature, congratulations—you're forest bathing!

Building familiarity with your "wild home" will deepen your forest therapy practice, so after you've chosen your "wild home," visit it as often as you can. Make sure you're comfortable and have water and maybe a snack with you, but that your phone is either left behind or on airplane mode to keep it from intruding. Then start walking, but channel your inner wide-eyed child and use your senses to really immerse yourself in the forest.

 ## Get a Green Thumb

Gardening can mean multiple raised beds in your backyard, or it can just mean a potted plant you keep on your windowsill. (Okay, windows are inside, but they still bring the outdoors in and therefore counts as outside.)

You can also get involved with a community garden in your area to learn more about gardening or just work on someone else's garden bed without committing 100% to your own.

Gardening is good for the planet (and can help counteract those climate change warnings that were probably flooding your feed before you did this detox), but it's also good for your physical and mental health, including many of the same benefits as forest therapy and of moderate exercise, but gardening might mean you also get fresh vegetables. Yum!

 Go Camping

Tents aren't just for scouts! Camping is one of the best ways to unplug for a significant amount of time. Take some friends, make some s'mores over a campfire, maybe take a hike if you're feeling extra bold, and you'll be shocked at how time flies when you're not engrossed in your phone. So what if Becky is in Cabo again? You're becoming one with nature and that's even better! (And just keep telling yourself that until you believe it.)

Or, if you're a camping pro and don't need anyone else there to pitch the tent for you, take a journal with you and really get in the mindfulness zone. If you don't want to invest a lot in camping gear, do some research and see if a local community group has any camping equipment that they rent or lend. Some libraries or community centers have tents or sleeping bags they lend for outdoor activities.

Get Sporty

If you love sports, then join a sports team so you get into a routine. If you're not so athletically inclined, pick a random sport you've never tried and just try it! You don't have to be great at tennis to work up a sweat, and you don't have to know basketball lingo to get outside with your kiddos and create family memories.

TAKE SOME "ME TIME"

It's important to invest in the person who should be your number one: yourself. You've probably/definitely heard about self-care; it's become a super trendy buzzword by now. But despite how you see it used online, it's not all about using bath bombs and dancing with no pants on (although both of those things help; we definitely still recommend them).

Self-care is the way you treat yourself every single day—so that includes the way you speak to yourself as well as the way you choose to spend your time. It's forgiving yourself the way you would your friends if they cancelled plans because they weren't in a great headspace. It's reminding yourself that you deserve more than a partner who won't call you back, the way you would your BFF.

It's making yourself a priority like you would your loved ones or your pets or your clients—or, hello, your phone. All those emails and notifications can wait. Your mental health cannot.

So spend some time with yourself! (If the sound of that makes you feel uncomfortable, guess what: That means you need to do it even more!) Get to know what really makes you happy, what doesn't, what you want out of life, and what you don't. Then adjust accordingly.

EXPRESS YOURSELF

 Journal it Out

There's no right or wrong way to journal. You can recap events and sort through your feelings, or you can start a daily gratitude log, you can write down fake letters to people you're mad at (to vent and, again, sort through your feelings), or you can make lists for what activities make you happy, who brings you joy (and what specific qualities they possess to bring about that joy), vacations you want to take, and books you want to read.

And we encourage you to journal throughout your digital detox (so much so that we've included puh-lenty of journaling pages for you later in this book). Journaling can really help you throughout your detoxes. You can document what you're giving up, why, for how long, your struggles and triumphs along the way, goals, and the final outcome. The great thing about documenting your digital detox through journaling is that you can really see your progress (or lack thereof), as well as your emotional journey.

 ## Channel Your Inner Jane Austen

Do you have stories rattling around in your brain? Or maybe when you're reading, you think of ways you'd rather the story go?

"JOURNALING IS LIKE HAVING A BEST FRIEND THAT YOU CAN SHARE EVERYTHING WITH ONLY THERE IS NO JUDGMENT."

–*Julee Hunt,* author of You Are Worthy: A Guide for the Overwhelmed Perfectionist

Consider flexing your creative writing muscle! Experiment with novel outlines, short story writing, or poetry. Create character outlines, and write down snippets of dialogue that you think of. If you like the ideas, keep working with them. If you don't like them, just move on to the next idea. No one has to see your ideas if you don't want them to!

 ## Unleash Your Inner Picasso

Getting creative has some major mental health benefits, so even if you're not so artistically inclined, try to at least give it your best shot. Whether you're interested in painting, photography, drawing Manga, or even just doodling, there's a class you can sign up for.

If you don't feel like you're classically artistic, check out crafting. Cross-stitch, crochet, and knitting, for example, are artsy hobbies, but there are many patterns available that a beginner can tackle, no problem. You can get started at your local craft store or with a how-to book.

CONNECT FOR REAL

A lot of the reasons we share so much on social media is because we're trying to form and maintain connections. So while you're detoxing, you'll need to make a concerted effort to stay connected to the people you care about the most.

 Phone a Friend

We know, we know, calling people is so early 2000s. But the longer you stick to your digital detox, the more you'll miss out on your friends' lives. Pick up the phone (yes, you're allowed to this time) and phone a friend. If you get super anxious making phone calls, set a timer. When it goes off, say your pet is dying to go outside or your dinner is done cooking. But make the most of every minute!

 Get Real Face Time

Better yet, visit your friend in person. Physical face time is so much better than digital FaceTime (get it?); bonus, your friend might even show you all the memes you're missing out on—it doesn't count as cheating because you won't be picking up your own phone to see them.

 Join a Club

Socializing with people who have similar interests will help you to keep your mind on other things during your digital detox. If you love to read, but have trouble sticking with a book until the end, a book club might help. After all, you have to finish it in order to discuss it with your friends.

Clubs also help you get involved in your community. In religious or political groups, you can talk about local issues with your neighbors and even volunteer together. (More on that next.)

Volunteer

Whether you're helping out at a soup kitchen, taking care of kitties and doggies at a shelter, cleaning up trash on the highway, or campaigning for your favorite local candidate, spending your free time volunteering will keep you grounded and remind you why you're detoxing in the first place. Being around other people (or furbabies) who aren't glued to a phone helps you to be more mindful of your technology usage.

If you aren't sure where to start, ask your friends or family if they know of any volunteer opportunities that would be a good fit. Your local library or newspaper are good sources for leads outside of your circle of friends, too. Chances are, there are dozens of organizations who would love a new energetic face.

HOW DID I "GO OUTSIDE?"

....

....

....

....

....

....

....

....

....

....

....

ASK YOURSELF

HOW DID I TAKE SOME "ME TIME?"

....

....

....

....

....

....

....

....

....

....

....

....

HOW DID I "EXPRESS MYSELF?"

....

....

....

....

....

....

....

....

....

....

....

....

HOW DID I "CONNECT FOR REAL?"

....

....

....

....

....

....

....

....

....

....

....

....

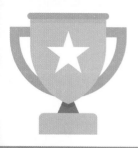

CHALLENGE

 ## GET OFF THE GRID

Up for a challenge? Don't just take a timeout from your devices; go dark for a full twenty-four hours. Totally unplug—that means no phone calls, no email, no text, no video games, no binge-watching anything. Make yourself as unreachable as possible and stay completely offline.

Think that sounds easy? Take it a step further and plan a camping trip or a stay in a rural cabin for a weekend. Adding nature into the mix will amplify the benefits of your digital vacation and not having a signal or a phone charger will help keep you honest.

(Note: If you're going to spend a weekend unreachable in the woods, make sure to tell a few people where you're going ahead of time, and make sure there's a reliable way to call emergency services, just in case something goes wrong!)

Tried it out? Tell us about it.

....

....

....

....

....

....

....

....

....

....

....

....

Maintenance Mode

Let's be real, you can't keep up the off-the-grid life forever. (At least, we can't.) That doesn't mean you have to have a full-blown backslide though! If you want to lose weight—and actually keep it off—you have to completely change your lifestyle as opposed to just dieting for a little while, right?

Well, the same principle applies here. To attain a healthy, balanced relationship with the digital technologies in your life, you have to make a few permanent changes. There are some steps you can take to maintain the ground you've gained.

🔔 **Keep all push notifications for social apps turned off.** Yes, we know, you don't want to miss a notification about your best friend tagging you in a meme. But once you've opened the app, you immediately get sucked into yet another endless scrolling session. Once you turn off push notifications, you'll realize how many notifications you get a day and be glad for the lack of distractions.

✉ **While you're at it, turn off notifications for your email.** Yes, even your work email. Notify people if you need to, but designate one or two specific times a day to responding to emails. You'd be amazed how much you can get done when you don't have emails popping up on your computer screen every fifteen minutes.

🗑 **Delete, delete, delete.** Keep your inbox decluttered by deleting unimportant emails, moving important ones into special folders, and unsubscribing from newsletters you never read.

🖥 **Make one room your digital zone.** And not the bedroom. Your bedroom should be a peaceful place; buy an alarm clock and charge your phone elsewhere.

🕐 **Download apps that track the amount of time you spend on the internet.** This will help you see which apps are sucking up most of your time, so you can adjust accordingly. You can also measure your progress during your digital detox and see the differences.

🍲 **Designate an hour (or more) each night to be technology-free.** And have a designed hobby to take its place, whether it's cooking dinner, reading a book, taking your dog for a walk, meditating, etc.

⊚ **Set goals each week for taking breaks from devices.** Start small! It's okay to start with a goal to only watch Netflix three days a week instead of seven. Remember, slow and steady wins the race.

🏋 **Decide what you want to do instead of being on your devices.** Read two books a month instead of binge-watching Netflix, or spend the two hours you usually spend on social media hitting the gym.

♥ **Forgive yourself.** If you slip up and watch Taylor Swift's newest music video on YouTube during a detox, guess what: you're human. (And Taylor Swift songs are annoyingly catchy, dang it.) Watch it another fifty-two times, get it out of your system, and then try, try again!

📈 **Track your progress.** It's easier to stay motivated if you can see your progress in front of you. We've provided a habit tracker in the following chapter.

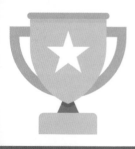

CHALLENGE

 APPLY THE POMODORO TECHNIQUE

Wait, what is the Pomodoro Technique? It's a time-management technique that was developed by Francesco Cirillo in the 1980s. Basically, it relies on setting short time periods for activities.

How can you apply this to your phone use? Set a timer for twenty-five minutes, and when the timer goes off you put your phone down and get back to work. The Pomodoro Technique is traditionally used for short bursts of productivity, but with a timer yelling at you to get off your phone, you're much more likely to do it! Use this whenever you get on your phone for a week. You can do this by buying a real timer (old school, right?) or simply by setting the timer on your phone.

Tried it out? Tell us about it.

....

....

....

....

....

....

....

....

....

....

....

....

....

....

....

....

....

....

Ready, Set, Detox

Now it's time to customize your very first Digital Detox Game Plan! Let's get down to the specifics of your digital detox. You'll need to decide a few things, like what you're giving up, for how long, what you're replacing technology with—the works.

This step is important because setting clear boundaries helps you stick to your guns and avoid cheating your way out of actually completing your detox through some loopholes. Instead of just writing out a whole list of what you're planning on cutting out for the detox, decide what's still going to be allowed. Maybe using a notes app on your tablet to make a grocery list is allowed, but no TV or movie streaming. Or Facebook isn't allowed, but LinkedIn is.

How long do you need to do a digital detox for it to really take effect? Rachel Anne Dine, LPC, recommends spending a solid ninety days free from technology. The first month is where you begin to try to break the habit of constantly checking social media or turning on Netflix as soon as you get home. Then the second month is where you start to find your equilibrium. "This may sound intense," Rachel says, "but you essentially have to recreate your life without social media." And the third month? That's where you'll really start to reap the benefits.

But reminder, it's okay to start small and work your way up to a ninety-day digital detox! If you're just starting out, Dr. Christopher Smithmyer, LLM, asserts that to break the cycle, you should do a digital detox for at least five days—this will give your body time to adjust to the lack of screen time. He says, "Do not be surprised if you feel stress or anxiety being away from your device, wondering 'what if someone is trying to reach me?'. There are other ways to reach you, it will be okay."

In the following worksheets, we'll give you a list of options for customizing your digital detoxes. This is **your** journey after all. We won't tell you how to reach the finish line; we'll simply provide you with the tools and guidance you need to do it yourself!

Once you've filled out your Digital Detox Game Plan, then you'll move on to the Habit Tracker. Here, you will write down any habits you think will support the success of your digital detox. Every day you successfully form (or break) that habit, you color in a little calendar block. Don't worry about being perfect; the main point of the Habit Tracker is to illustrate the progress you've made on your journey so far.

"WE NEED TO FIND A BALANCE WHERE WE'RE NOT COMPLETELY UNPLUGGED, BUT WE'RE ALSO NOT SOLELY RELIANT ON DIGITAL TOOLS."

—*Lisa Chau*, Digital Strategist, published in *Forbes, Buzzfeed, Thrive Global, US News & World Report,* and *Huffington Post*

DIGITAL DETOX GAME PLAN

For   1   2   3   4   5   6   7   8

9   10   11   12   13   14   15   16

17   18   19   20   21   22   23   24

25   26   27   28   29   30   31

days / weeks / month
(circle one)

I'm giving up...

- ☐ Facebook
- ☐ Instagram
- ☐ Twitter
- ☐ Phone
- ☐ Netflix
- ☐ Hulu
- ☐ Cable
- ☐ Amazon Prime
- ☐ HBO Now
- ☐ ....
- ☐ ....
- ☐ ....

I'll use my new found free time to

....

....

....

....

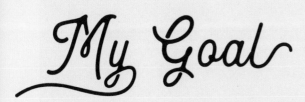

My Goal

What do I hope to achieve by digital detoxing?

....
....
....
....
....
....
....
....
....
....
....

Habit Tracker

HABIT 1

1	2	3	4	5	6	7	8	9	10	11	12	13	14
16	17	18	19	20	21	22	23	24	25	26	27	28	29	30

HABIT 3

1	2	3	4	5	6	7	8	9	10	11	12	13	14
16	17	18	19	20	21	22	23	24	25	26	27	28	29	30

HABIT 5

1	2	3	4	5	6	7	8	9	10	11	12	13	14
16	17	18	19	20	21	22	23	24	25	26	27	28	29	30

HABIT 7

1	2	3	4	5	6	7	8	9	10	11	12	13	14
16	17	18	19	20	21	22	23	24	25	26	27	28	29	30

ABIT 2

| 2 | 3 | 4 | 5 | 6 | 7 | 8 | 9 | 10 | 11 | 12 | 13 | 14 | 15 |
| 17 | 18 | 19 | 20 | 21 | 22 | 23 | 24 | 25 | 26 | 27 | 28 | 29 | 30 | 31 |

ABIT 4

| 2 | 3 | 4 | 5 | 6 | 7 | 8 | 9 | 10 | 11 | 12 | 13 | 14 | 15 |
| 17 | 18 | 19 | 20 | 21 | 22 | 23 | 24 | 25 | 26 | 27 | 28 | 29 | 30 | 31 |

ABIT 6

| 2 | 3 | 4 | 5 | 6 | 7 | 8 | 9 | 10 | 11 | 12 | 13 | 14 | 15 |
| 17 | 18 | 19 | 20 | 21 | 22 | 23 | 24 | 25 | 26 | 27 | 28 | 29 | 30 | 31 |

ABIT 8

| 2 | 3 | 4 | 5 | 6 | 7 | 8 | 9 | 10 | 11 | 12 | 13 | 14 | 15 |
| 17 | 18 | 19 | 20 | 21 | 22 | 23 | 24 | 25 | 26 | 27 | 28 | 29 | 30 | 31 |

DIGITAL DETOX GAME PLAN

For   1   2   3   4   5   6   7   8

       9   10 11 12 13 14 15 16

    17 18 19 20 21 22 23 24

    25 26 27 28 29 30 31   days / weeks / month
                                          (circle one)

I'm giving up...

- [ ] Facebook
- [ ] Instagram
- [ ] Twitter
- [ ] Phone
- [ ] Netflix
- [ ] Hulu
- [ ] Cable
- [ ] Amazon Prime
- [ ] HBO Now
- [ ] ....
- [ ] ....
- [ ] ....

I'll use my new found free time to

....

....

....

....

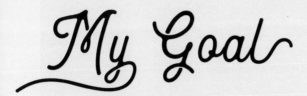

My Goal

What do I hope to achieve by digital detoxing?

....

....

....

....

....

....

....

....

....

....

....

Habit Tracker

HABIT 1

1	2	3	4	5	6	7	8	9	10	11	12	13	14	1
16	17	18	19	20	21	22	23	24	25	26	27	28	29	30	

HABIT 3

1	2	3	4	5	6	7	8	9	10	11	12	13	14	1
16	17	18	19	20	21	22	23	24	25	26	27	28	29	30	

HABIT 5

1	2	3	4	5	6	7	8	9	10	11	12	13	14	1
16	17	18	19	20	21	22	23	24	25	26	27	28	29	30	

HABIT 7

1	2	3	4	5	6	7	8	9	10	11	12	13	14	1
16	17	18	19	20	21	22	23	24	25	26	27	28	29	30	

HABIT 2

| | 2 | 3 | 4 | 5 | 6 | 7 | 8 | 9 | 10 | 11 | 12 | 13 | 14 | 15 |
| | 17 | 18 | 19 | 20 | 21 | 22 | 23 | 24 | 25 | 26 | 27 | 28 | 29 | 30 | 31 |

HABIT 4

| | 2 | 3 | 4 | 5 | 6 | 7 | 8 | 9 | 10 | 11 | 12 | 13 | 14 | 15 |
| | 17 | 18 | 19 | 20 | 21 | 22 | 23 | 24 | 25 | 26 | 27 | 28 | 29 | 30 | 31 |

HABIT 6

| | 2 | 3 | 4 | 5 | 6 | 7 | 8 | 9 | 10 | 11 | 12 | 13 | 14 | 15 |
| | 17 | 18 | 19 | 20 | 21 | 22 | 23 | 24 | 25 | 26 | 27 | 28 | 29 | 30 | 31 |

HABIT 8

| | 2 | 3 | 4 | 5 | 6 | 7 | 8 | 9 | 10 | 11 | 12 | 13 | 14 | 15 |
| | 17 | 18 | 19 | 20 | 21 | 22 | 23 | 24 | 25 | 26 | 27 | 28 | 29 | 30 | 31 |

DIGITAL DETOX GAME PLAN

For 1   2   3   4   5   6   7   8
     9   10 11 12 13 14 15 16
     17 18 19 20 21 22 23 24
     25 26 27 28 29 30 31   days / weeks / month
                                          (circle one)

I'm giving up...
- ☐ Facebook
- ☐ Instagram
- ☐ Twitter
- ☐ Phone
- ☐ Netflix
- ☐ Hulu
- ☐ Cable
- ☐ Amazon Prime
- ☐ HBO Now
- ☐ ....
- ☐ ....
- ☐ ....

I'll use my new found free time to

....

....

....

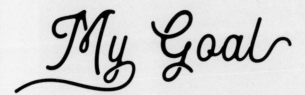

My Goal

What do I hope to achieve by digital detoxing?

....

....

....

....

....

....

....

....

....

....

....

Habit Tracker

HABIT 1

| 1 | 2 | 3 | 4 | 5 | 6 | 7 | 8 | 9 | 10 | 11 | 12 | 13 | 14 | 15 |
| 16 | 17 | 18 | 19 | 20 | 21 | 22 | 23 | 24 | 25 | 26 | 27 | 28 | 29 | 30 | |

HABIT 3

| 1 | 2 | 3 | 4 | 5 | 6 | 7 | 8 | 9 | 10 | 11 | 12 | 13 | 14 | 15 |
| 16 | 17 | 18 | 19 | 20 | 21 | 22 | 23 | 24 | 25 | 26 | 27 | 28 | 29 | 30 | 3 |

HABIT 5

| 1 | 2 | 3 | 4 | 5 | 6 | 7 | 8 | 9 | 10 | 11 | 12 | 13 | 14 | 15 |
| 16 | 17 | 18 | 19 | 20 | 21 | 22 | 23 | 24 | 25 | 26 | 27 | 28 | 29 | 30 | 3 |

HABIT 7

| 1 | 2 | 3 | 4 | 5 | 6 | 7 | 8 | 9 | 10 | 11 | 12 | 13 | 14 | 15 |
| 16 | 17 | 18 | 19 | 20 | 21 | 22 | 23 | 24 | 25 | 26 | 27 | 28 | 29 | 30 | 3 |

MONTH:

ABIT 2

| 2 | 3 | 4 | 5 | 6 | 7 | 8 | 9 | 10 | 11 | 12 | 13 | 14 | 15 |
| 17 | 18 | 19 | 20 | 21 | 22 | 23 | 24 | 25 | 26 | 27 | 28 | 29 | 30 | 31 |

ABIT 4

| 2 | 3 | 4 | 5 | 6 | 7 | 8 | 9 | 10 | 11 | 12 | 13 | 14 | 15 |
| 17 | 18 | 19 | 20 | 21 | 22 | 23 | 24 | 25 | 26 | 27 | 28 | 29 | 30 | 31 |

ABIT 6

| 2 | 3 | 4 | 5 | 6 | 7 | 8 | 9 | 10 | 11 | 12 | 13 | 14 | 15 |
| 17 | 18 | 19 | 20 | 21 | 22 | 23 | 24 | 25 | 26 | 27 | 28 | 29 | 30 | 31 |

ABIT 8

| 2 | 3 | 4 | 5 | 6 | 7 | 8 | 9 | 10 | 11 | 12 | 13 | 14 | 15 |
| 17 | 18 | 19 | 20 | 21 | 22 | 23 | 24 | 25 | 26 | 27 | 28 | 29 | 30 | 31 |

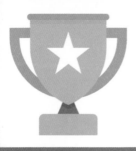

CHALLENGE

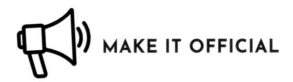 **MAKE IT OFFICIAL**

Unless you plan on straight-up ghosting your friends and followers, you should figure out how you want to tell people about your detox plans. You *could* call everyone in your contacts list, or you can use social media to let everyone know in one fell swoop. Below, we've drafted up a digital detox announcement to get you started. Now it's time to make it your own.

The Short and Sweet Announcement:

"Long story short, I've decided to take a short break from social media. If you need to get in touch with me in the next [X days/ weeks/months], call me or talk to me in person!"

Tried it out? Tell us about it.

....

....

....

....

....

....

....

....

....

....

....

....

....

....

Journal it Out

If you're tempted to skip this chapter because you don't like journaling or just because you're getting close to the end of the book, don't! Whatever kind of digital detox you choose to do, one thing is for sure: You need to journal about it. We covered this earlier, but keeping a journal can be your secret digital detoxing weapon because of the way it engages different parts of your brain, and helps you work through emotion.

Maybe you've tried to journal before, and didn't like it. Or you actually enjoyed journaling, but still struggled to make it a habit. That's okay—journaling isn't one-size fits all! There are different ways to journal.

STREAM-OF-CONSCIOUSNESS JOURNALING

If you've given up on journaling in the past because you can't quiet your inner critic telling you to correct your grammar or write something more original, give stream of consciousness journaling a try. Laura Rhodes-Levin recommends stream-of-conciousness journaling specifically for digital detoxing to process your thoughts and feelings about any difficulty you're experiencing. "Just let your hand move freely with any thought that comes to your mind," she suggests, "letting go of the need to create any specific order to what you are writing."

When you're starting out with stream-of-consciousness journaling, it can be helpful to set a short timer and dedicate yourself to writing for at least five minutes (but of course, you can continue if you're in the mood!).

GRATITUDE JOURNALING

Susan Petang, a certified mindful lifestyle and stress management coach and author of *The Quiet Zone: Mindful Stress Management for Everyday People*, has found that a gratitude log is a valuable transformation tool. She says, "The physical act of writing creates neural pathways in our brains, cementing the information so that we retain it better. The same applies to writing down instances for which we can be grateful." Ever heard of the domino effect? The more you practice gratitude—no matter how small or inconsequential these things may seem—the more things and people and moments you will notice you're grateful for.

Gratitude journaling is a nice way to dip your toe into the journaling world. It's a good entry point because it's a focused type of journaling, and it's a quick way to start building a more positive outlook on your life. If you've tried journaling before, but didn't enjoy it because a blank page seemed overwhelming, gratitude journaling might be more your speed.

"GRATITUDE JOURNALING
CAN TURN ANY NEGATIVE
INTO A POSITIVE BECAUSE
IT'S IMPOSSIBLE TO BE
NEGATIVE AND GRATEFUL
AT THE SAME TIME."

–*Julee Hunt*, Worthiness Expert

NAME THREE THINGS YOU'RE GRATEFUL FOR EVERY NIGHT FOR A WEEK.

DAY: ....

1. ....

2. ....

3. ....

DAY: ....

1. ....

2. ....

3. ....

DAY: ....

1. ....

2. ....

3. ....

DAY: ....

1. ....

2. ....

3. ....

DAY: ....

1. ....

2. ....

3. ....

DAY: ....

1. ....

2. ....

3. ....

DAY: ....

1. ....

2. ....

3. ....

GRATITUDE JOURNALING

NAME THREE THINGS YOU'RE GRATEFUL FOR EVERY NIGHT FOR A WEEK.

DAY: ....

1. ....

2. ....

3. ....

DAY: ....

1. ....

2. ....

3. ....

DAY: ....

1. ....

2. ....

3. ....

DAY: ....

1. ....

2. ....

3. ....

DAY: ....

1. ....

2. ....

3. ....

DAY: ....

1. ....

2. ....

3. ....

DAY: ....

1. ....

2. ....

3. ....

GRATITUDE JOURNALING

NAME THREE THINGS YOU'RE GRATEFUL FOR EVERY NIGHT FOR A WEEK.

DAY: ....

1. ....

2. ....

3. ....

DAY: ....

1. ....

2. ....

3. ....

DAY: ....

1. ....

2. ....

3. ....

DAY: ....
1. ....
....
2. ....
....
3. ....

DAY: ....
1. ....
....
2. ....
....
3. ....

DAY: ....
1. ....
....
2. ....
....
3. ....

DAY: ....
1. ....
....
2. ....
....
3. ....

GRATITUDE JOURNALING

HAVE YOU NOTICED ANY CHANGES IN YOUR MOOD
OR BEHAVIOR SINCE YOU BEGAN GRATITUDE
JOURNALING?

....

....

....

....

....

....

....

LOOK BACK AT YOUR LISTS. WRITE THREE WORDS
THAT DESCRIBE HOW THE LISTS MAKE YOU FEEL.

1. ....

2. ....

3. ....

ART JOURNALING

Art journaling is the practice of visually representing your thoughts, feelings, and ideas. If expressing yourself in writing doesn't come naturally to you, it might help to try art journaling. On the flip side, if expressing yourself artistically doesn't come naturally, art journaling is a great way to reconnect to your creative side.

Like you would with any other journaling practice, set aside some time each day for your art journal. Then draw, doodle, or write whatever you want! You can even include pictures you've taken, or cut out images from magazines to help you express yourself. Your journal pages can be as elaborate or as simple as you like.

In the following pages, we have added several prompts to get your creative juices flowing. Not your style? Just record any struggles you're having, your successes, how good it feels to live in the moment, etc. Record every detail so you can 1.) look back at your progress, and 2.) remember how worth it it was. Digital detoxing is kind of like going to the gym; you dread it (obviously), but afterwards, the endorphins kick in and you feel like you could take over the world.

If you don't have a whole lot of time to journal, or you don't consider yourself much of a journaler, keep it simple and record the key takeaways from your day or week. It doesn't even have to be longer than a sentence.

Now you're on your own, but you've made it this far so you're going to be just fine. Before we cut you loose, there are some writing prompts to help you get in the journaling rhythm. Like everything else in this book, if these prompts don't resonate with you, then ignore them and write about whatever you want.

"JOURNAL ABOUT YOUR EMOTIONAL STATE, A HIGH POINT OF THE DAY, AND LOW POINT, AND THEN REFER BACK TO IT AND FIND THE COMMON LINKS; LIKE, 'EVERY MONDAY I HAVE SEVERE ANXIETY.' IT'S JUST A GOOD TOOL TO BE ABLE TO GO BACK TO BECAUSE IT INCREASES YOUR SELF-AWARENESS."

—Rachel Anne Dine, LPC

After I check social media, I feel:

....

....

....

....

....

....

....

....

....

....

....

....

....

....

....

....

....

....

....

....

My life summed up in movie titles is:

1. ....
....
....
....

2. ....
....
....

3. ....
....
....
....

I feel the most connected to my friends when I:

....

....

....

....

....

....

....

....

....

....

....

....

I've discovered that I am my most mindful when:

....

....

....

....

....

....

....

....

....

....

....

It is important to me to connect with:

....

....

....

....

....

....

....

....

....

....

Three people who have influenced me are:

1. ....
....
....
....

2. ....
....
....
....

3. ....
....
....
....

If my life were a song, it would be:

....

....

....

....

....

....

....

....

....

....

....

If I could meet anyone, it would be:

....

....

....

....

....

....

....

....

....

....

....

A tough time that I overcame was:

....

....

....

....

....

....

....

....

....

....

....

....

If I were an animal, I'd be:

....

....

....

....

....

....

....

....

....

....

....

A perfect day would be:

....

....

....

....

....

....

....

....

....

....

....

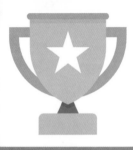

CHALLENGE

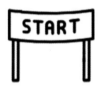

TRY SOMETHING NEW

Some of these are probably brand-new journaling techniques for you (and it's easy to skip out on new and unfamiliar things), so we're challenging you to try each one! You might find something you really love.

If none of these are new for you, then go one step farther and try to think of a creative way you can approach journaling on your own. Talk with your friends to see if they have a journaling technique that they really love. If that's a dead end, look to your favorite book or movie character for inspiration, or even try your hand at writing a poem or a (very) short story.

Tried it out? Tell us about it.

ACKNOWLEDGMENTS

Infinite thanks to the experts who took the time to help us out: Julee Hunt, Worthiness Expert and author of *You Are Worthy: A Guide For The Overwhelmed Perfectionist*; Amos Clifford, founder of the Association of Nature and Forest Therapy and author of *Your Guide to Forest Bathing*; Vicki Yaffe, certified life coach; Rachel Anne Dine, Licensed Professional Counselor (LPC), owner of Humanitas Counseling and Consulting; Lisa Chau, founder of Alpha Vert, a private consultancy focused on social media and cross-platform marketing; Laura Rhodes-Levin, Licensed Marriage and Family Therapist (LMFT) and founder of The Missing Peace Center for Anxiety; Susan Petang, author of *The Quiet Zone: Mindful Stress Management for Everyday People*; and Melanie Choukas-Bradley, naturalist and author of *The Joy of Forest Bathing: Reconnect With Wild Places & Rejuvenate Your Life.*

Our significant others have been angling for a book mention, so here is where we're going to thank them as well as the amazing friends and family that come together to form a robust support system. Thank you for being there for us during the late nights, encouraging us when writing wasn't coming naturally, and believing in us every step of the way.

ABOUT THE AUTHORS

ELISE WILLIAMS RIKARD

Elise Williams Rikard is an editor and co-author of *Common Cents* and *You Goal, Girl*—but when binge-watching Sailor Moon and eating frozen pizza becomes a profitable career, she'll leave the publishing world behind. She has a BA in technical writing from the University of Central Arkansas and lives in Arkansas with her husband Cody and her cat Lazarus.

MELEAH BOWLES

Meleah Bowles co-founded Earn Spend Live and co-authored *Common Cents* and *You Goal, Girl*. Despite her weird preoccupation with making a "Twenty in their Twenties" list, she is really fun at parties (pinky promise). She lives in Arkansas with her partner and their two dogs. She has a BA in technical writing from the University of Central Arkansas.

RESOURCES

Barton, Jo & Pretty, Jules. "What is the Best Dose of Nature and Green Exercise for Improving Mental Health? A Multi-Study Analysis." Environmental Science & Technology, vol. 44, no. 10, 2010, pp. 3947-55, doi: 3947-55. 10.1021/es903183r.

Centers for Disease Control and Prevention (CDC). "Perceived Insufficient Rest or Sleep among Adults - United States, 2008." Morbidity and Mortality Weekly Report, vol. 58, no. 42, 30 Oct. 2008.

Chau, Lisa. Personal Interview. 26 Apr. 2019.

Choukas-Bradley, Melanie. The Joy of Forest Bathing: Reconnect With Wild Places & Rejuvenate Your Life. Rock Point, 4 Sept. 2018.

Clifford, Amos. Personal Interview. 30 Apr. 2019.

Dine, Rachel Anne. Personal interview. 1 May 2019.

Hunt, Julee. Personal Interview. 3 May 2019.

Klepeis, Neil E, et al. "The National Human Activity Pattern Survey (NHAPS): a Resource for Assessing Exposure to Environmental Pollutants." Journal of Exposure Science & Environmental Epidemiology, vol. 11, no. 3, 26 July 2001, pp. 231-252., doi:10.1038/sj.jea.7500165.

Ledger of Harms. Center for Humane Technology, 14 Dec. 2018, ledger.humanetech.com/.

Mangen, Anne, and Jean-Luc Velay. "Digitizing Literacy: Reflections on the Haptics of Writing." Advances in Haptics, edited by Mehrdad Hosseini Zadeh, IntechOpen, 2010.

Petang, Susan. Personal interview. 3 May 2019.

Przybylski, Andrew K., and Netta Weinstein. "Can You Connect with Me Now? How the Presence of Mobile Communication Technology Influences Face-to-Face Conversation Quality." Journal of Social and Personal Relationships, vol. 30, no. 3, May 2013, pp. 237-246, doi:10.1177/0265407512453827.

Rhodes-Levin, Laura. Personal Interview. 28 Apr. 2019.

Smithmyer, Christopher. Personal interview. 27 Apr. 2019.

Wurmser, Yoram. "Mobile Time Spent 2018." EMarketer, 18 June 2018, www.emarketer.com/content/mobile-time-spent-2018.

Yaffe, Vikki. Personal interview. 20 Apr. 2019.